FOOD

FOR

LIFE:

A Day-at-a-Time Guide

FOOD
FOR
LIFE:

A Day-at-a-Time Guide

Pamela M. Smith, R.D.

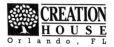

CREATION
HOUSE
Orlando, FL

FOOD FOR LIFE: A DAY-AT-A-TIME GUIDE
Published by Creation House
Strang Communications Company
600 Rinehart Road
Lake Mary, Florida 32746
Web site: http://www.creationhouse.com

Unless otherwise noted, all Scripture quotations are from
the Holy Bible, New International Version. Copyright © 1973,
1978, 1984, International Bible Society. Used by permission.

Scripture quotations marked KJV are from the King James
Version of the Bible.

CONTENTS

❖ ❖ ❖

LEADER'S GUIDE / 73

INTRODUCTION

Welcome to this devotional study guide, which accompanies Pam Smith's best-selling book, *Food For Life*. This devotional guide is written for individuals or small groups who wish to probe more deeply into Bible study, interact with the content of the book, and share accountably with others the truths discovered here for healthy eating and living.

Four guides for groups or class sessions are at the end of this study for use by group leaders or teachers. Groups using this guide should complete their assigned devotional studies and readings in the book prior to their group sessions. This will greatly enhance sharing, study, and praying together.

Individuals using this guide can use it for daily devotional reading and study. Keep a daily journal to jot down your notes, thoughts, and log your eating pattern. By journaling your thoughts and activities, you will notice the change in your eating habits and lifestyle as a result of applying God's Word and this study guide to your life. Each daily devotional study is structured to aid you to:

▲ Encounter God's Word.
▲ Complete assigned reading and action steps from *Food For Life*.
▲ Embrace life-giving principles and affirmations for developing a healthy lifestyle.

▲ Be set free from rationalizations, food traps, and unhealthy eating habits.

We pray that this study guide will be an effective tool for equipping you to live better and longer through the nourishing of your body, soul, and spirit. You will find that food, though physical, reflects spiritual issues. Be prepared to examine your own eating and living habits through this light. Approach these issues prayerfully, asking for truth to be revealed to you. You may want to offer this prayer before and after you do each lesson:

Lord, change my heart, and let that change be revealed in my life. Amen.

L IVING W ELL

*But I will restore you to health and heal your
wounds, declares the Lord.*
                                    —JEREMIAH 30:17

D o you fully understand that God wants you well?
That He intends for His children to value themselves and to walk in the purpose for which He
created them? It's true—we were created with health
and healing scripted into every cell of our bodies. We
only need to embrace that truth—and to learn to live life
in such a way as to release, not block, that flow of
healing to get well and stay well. Then taking care of
ourselves flows out of a natural desire to be healthy and
happy, not out of duty or feelings of guilt. And as we
live well, it overflows into those around us.

Yet, too many of us don't live well. We get caught in
the snares of life—lack of self-care, erratic eating,
unhealthy choices, poor sleep patterns, no exercise—all
hindering abundant living. We need a new perspective
on food—physical, emotional, and spiritual food—that
frees us to be well and energizes us to live fulfilled lives.

I pray that this week will be one in which you will be
encouraged with hope, truth, and practical helps for dis-
covering the life of wellness planned for you.

ACTION STEP FOR WEEK 1:

Keep a diary of everything you eat and drink, the time
that you eat, how you are feeling, and any exercise you
may do (see sample and blank diaries on pages 41–43 of

Food for Life). As you keep track of how you are living each day, look for the areas that may be contributing to your body's not working at its best.

VISION STATEMENT

This week you will embrace the truth that God wants you well, and will receive His healing power in every area of your life. You are empowered to be spiritually strong, to be emotionally strong and stable, to have a strong and healthy body, and to enjoy a healthy relationship with God, yourself, others, and food.

Day 1

[Read pages 9–14 of *Food For Life*.]

LIVING LIFE TODAY

I can do everything through him who gives me strength.

—PHILIPPIANS 4:13

Today's lifestyle requires energy—lots of it. Everyone dreams of living a full life and feeling great. Wellness has become a byword of our culture. Most of us do not need to know how to diet or control disease, but how to eat for a healthy life in which we can enjoy all that God has for us physically, emotionally, mentally, and spiritually.

Step back for a moment and look at yourself. There is more to living well than just caring for and feeding your physical being. You need to care for and feed your soul with the right kind of soul food. Look at the following statements and underline all those that fit you:

▲ I am out of energy and out of control, especially with my health and eating.
▲ I am caught in a food trap of overeating, dieting, and watching my weight.
▲ I find myself underfed and underfueled.
▲ I am too busy or too tired to do anything about what I eat or how I take care of myself.
▲ I feed my body but not my soul.
▲ I am too exhausted at the end of the day to do anything but zone out.
▲ I don't have extra energy when I need it for doing things I enjoy.

3

This study will help you remove the logjams to your physical and emotional well-being so that you will release a virtual river of abundant life and energy.

In what areas do you need to increase your energy for life? Below are some energy gauges from empty to full that represent each area of your life. Put an x on the line that represents where you are right now.

1. My physical energy for life is _____
   Empty   Full
2. My emotional energy for life is_____
   Empty   Full
3. My mental energy for life is _____
   Empty   Full
4. My spiritual energy for life is_____
   Empty   Full

ASSESSING YOUR DAY

- ▲ How do you usually feel when you wake up in the morning?_____
- ▲ Do you often experience physical or emotional rises and falls throughout your day?_____
- ▲ Are there times when hunger or cravings seem to overtake you?_____ When?_____
- ▲ How do you satisfy that hunger?_____
- ▲ How do you sleep at night? _____

ASK GOD . . .

To give you the strength and focus you need to be honest about your daily eating and living habits—and to illuminate any rationalizations that you may have been using to justify your eating habits.

4

[Read pages 20–24 of *Food For Life.*]

STOP DIETING, START LIVING

It is for freedom that Christ has set us free. Stand firm, then, and do not let yourselves be burdened again by a yoke of slavery.

—GALATIANS 5:1

A woman once told me, "I'm forty-something and feel as if I've been fighting a war against my body for forty-some years. I just can't lose weight and keep it off. I think I've tried every diet created. I've swallowed pills, taken shots, and eaten formulated foods and powders. I've fasted and drunk protein shakes. I've prayed and been prayed for."

I see people every day who desire, maybe obsessively, a thin and healthy body, but such a body seems to be an impossible dream. The odds are an overwhelming nine to one that people who have lost weight will gain it back within a year. How about you? (Put an *x* on the line.)

I desire to lose _____ pounds and keep it off.

_____

Somewhat   Moderately   Intensely

When I diet, I usually put most of the weight back on after:

_____

1 month   6 months   1 year

Until we are ready to be set free from a dieting mindset and embark on a lifestyle of health, then sickness, fatigue, lack of self-care, overeating, or weight can have a powerful grip on our lives.

In your own words, explain the difference between "going on a diet" and "eating for life."

_____

_____

_____

PERSONAL INVENTORY

Where would I like to be in the area of:

My health _____

My energy _____

My appearance _____

My muscle tone _____

My weight _____

My clothing size _____

My fitness level _____

Read the following scriptures, and jot down what they say about your thought life:

▲ Proverbs 23:7 _____

▲ 2 Corinthians 10:3–5 _____

▲ Philippians 3:19 _____

▲ 1 Corinthians 15:32 _____

Look clearly at your dieting experience. Do you see anything wrong with your picture? If you've been trying and failing for many years, it's not that you don't have enough willpower or discipline. Have you ever considered that you are choosing the wrong way to go about it? It's not that you need to learn _how to diet;_ instead you need to learn _how to eat for life._

Read what Jesus says about food and life in John 6:1–15 and 22–40. In your journal, summarize what He is saying to you about food and life.

ASK GOD . . .

To transform you by the renewing of your mind (Rom. 12:1–2). Ask Him to reveal the areas in which you have "conformed to the dieting ways and unhealthy beliefs of this world" and to set in place healthy truths about your body, food, and eating. Ask Him to give you the desire to eat well, live well.

[Read pages 24–26 of *Food For Life.*]

TAKE HOLD OF FREEDOM

I am the bread of life. He who comes to me will never go hungry, and he who believes in me will never be thirsty.

—JOHN 6:35

People feel guilty about eating unhealthy, "bad" food. They are constantly at war within themselves over doing what's right, or reverting to unhealthy desires. In the area of food, their biggest mistake is not what they eat; it's what they *don't* eat.

The key to healthy eating is having the right perspective. The fact is that eating well is a precious gift you give to yourself. It focuses on the fresh, flavorful, and fun foods that give the body energy and health—and give you better moods!

Food is an ally, not an enemy to be feared. Are you fighting a war with food? Here is a self-test to help you determine just how serious your war with food may be. Answer *Y* for *yes* or *N* for *no* to each of the following questions:

_____ Do you make promises to control your eating but break those promises again and again?

_____ Do you regularly go the whole day with little or no food, yet wonder why you are sick and tired?

_____ Do you deny the physical damage or complications caused by your eating choices?

_____ Are you constantly dieting or discussing food and weight loss?

_____ Are you driven by the desire to be thin, equating thinness with success and being in control?

_____ Do you eat more, or at a more frenzied pace, when under stress?

_____ Have you ever thought, *I was bad today; I'll starve myself tomorrow?*

_____ Do you binge the week before going on a diet?

_____ Have you eaten to the point of nausea, vomiting, or until your stomach hurts?

_____ Do others view your shape differently than you do?

_____ Do you eat when you feel good, or do you eat to relieve negative feelings?

_____ Do you avoid social engagements that involve eating if you are on a diet?

_____ Do you fast or drastically cut and count calories to lose weight?

_____ Do you have an on-a-diet, off-a-diet mentality, rather than eating moderately and wisely as the norm?

_____ Do you think of food as bad or forbidden rather than simply as food?

_____ Do you try to lose weight to look good for someone else?

_____ Have you relied on diet pills or shakes or any product that promises to do the weight-loss work for you?

_____ Do you try to lose weight with the mind-set that when you shed unwanted pounds, you will become a wonderful person, forgetting that you already are a wonderful person?

If you answered *yes* to a number of these, then the daily food fight has taken on a life of its own. Pick the top three issues you struggle with on the list and write them again, personalizing them:

1. I _____
_____.

2. I _____
_____.

3. I _____
_____.

Read what Jesus says about food and life in John 6:1–15 and 22–40. Summarize in your journal what He is saying about the role of food in your own life.

ASK GOD . . .

To change your perspective from "living to eat" to "eating to live." Ask Jesus for His bread that satisfies. Believe for the strength to let food be food, and God be God.

Day 4

[Read pages 28–30 of *Food For Life*.]

NOURISHING THE WHOLE BEING

The eyes of all look to you, and you give them their food at the proper time. You open your hand and satisfy the desires of every living thing.

—PSALM 145:15

We humans are three-part beings—body, soul, and spirit—and have needs to be nourished. Caring for the whole being means that we do special things to develop and maintain the health and inherent potential of all three arenas of ourselves. We oftentimes stumble because we don't get our needs met on all three levels, or because our lifestyle choices logjam the flow of abundant life.

Yet we often find ourselves doing the very things we hate. Well, here too we have good company! The apostle Paul wrote of this struggle: "I do not understand what I do. For what I want to do I do not do, but what I hate I do" (Rom. 7:15). Paul's spirit was born again and all things had become new. But his soul—mind and emotions—was clothed in the old.

It's not always easy to change habits and consistently do what is right. But it is possible. Expect resistance. Habits and thought patterns that have been learned throughout a lifetime require supernatural power and patience to unlearn.

Do you have areas in which you are being robbed? Do you see your health, your eating habits, or your attitudes about weight, food, or dieting affecting you in these areas?

11

▲ Your self-esteem   yes   no
▲ Your relationship with God   yes   no
▲ Your relationship with others   yes   no
▲ Your job, school, career   yes   no

I have a word for you: You don't have to push or drag through each day. You can have abundant life (John 10:10) and take charge of your own wellness, your energy level, and your weight. And you can be set free from the following traps that bind you to old habits. Which of the following traps do you need to be set free from?

❑ Overeating
❑ Stress
❑ Too little rest
❑ Constant dieting
❑ Bad attitudes about food
❑ Going long hours without eating
❑ Little or no exercise

With God's help you can be set free from these traps. Choose to look to Him for the food that gives life.

ASK GOD . . .

To allow you to see clearly the life traps that are robbing you of life—and to set you free from these traps that hinder your walk in abundant living.

12

[Read pages 30–31 of *Food For Life.*]

FREE TO BE WELL

Then you will know the truth, and the truth will set you free.

—JOHN 8:32

Before I embraced nutrition as a profession, I was handicapped in all three areas of my life—spirit, soul, and body. I was searching for real answers to my questions about the purpose of my life.

Put an *x* on the line where you identify:

▲ The purpose of my life is _____.
                       clear to me   a mystery
▲ My goals for this year are _____.
                       clear to me   a mystery
▲ Spiritually I am _____.
                   connected   in a vacuum
▲ Mentally and emotionally I am _____.
                       stable   confused
▲ Physically I am _____.
              strong and well   sick and tired
▲ Besides God, the person(s)
  I am accountable to are _____.
              strong and caring   nonexistent

When I asked tough questions of myself, I knew I was spiritually empty, but I didn't have a clue about how to get filled. I was carrying a lot of emotional baggage. Food became the obvious way to fill up my vacuums; it was also the fuel I used to carry my emotional burdens.

So I was trapped—emotionally, spiritually, and physically.

Indicate the traps you are facing in each of the following areas of your life.

BODY

SOUL   SPIRIT

As I learned more about nutrition and began to take care of my physical body, I became strong enough to overcome many of my unhealthy eating patterns.

Whatever our need of the moment—losing weight, gaining weight, controlling overeating, getting well—the goal is to learn how to get the body working *for* us and *with* us.

The Bible teaches that our bodies are the temple of the Holy Spirit (1 Cor. 3:16). Make it an important priority in your life to care for your temple.

ASK GOD . . .

To show you clear ways to care for your body, soul, and spirit—and to give you the determination and courage to set goals to do so.

Day 6

[Read pages 32–36 of *Food For Life*.]

Fuel the Power

*He gives strength to the weary and increases the
power of the weak . . . those who hope in the Lord
will renew their strength.*

—Isaiah 40:29, 31

In recent years I have counseled many professional
athletes, teaching them to "fuel the power," to be the
very best they can be—to win! My goal is to help
them operate from a point of physical strength, allowing
their natural gifts and learned skills to flow freely. My
goal as a nutritionist is to get the players' bodies strong
and stable. To win consistently, athletes have to stay
properly fit and fueled. The same is true for all of us.

From working with athletes, as well as with my other
clients, I have observed seven secrets for staying fit and
fueled. By following these secrets, you can embrace a
fulfilled and effective lifestyle—"fueling the power."

The seven food-for-life secrets are not a magic formula
to follow—they are timeless truths that demonstrate how
the body was designed to work, and how to make food,
exercise, and rest work for you, not against you.

Under each of the seven secrets listed below, place an
x on the line to represent where you are right now:

The Seven Secrets for Staying Fit, Fueled, and Free

1. *Eating is better than starving.* Eat early. Eat often. Eat
   balanced. Eat lean.

Never do this   Always do this

15

2. *Water is the beverage of champions.* Drink eight to ten eight-ounce servings of water each day

Never do this   Always do this

3. *Variety is the spice of life.* Include a healthy variety of foods in your daily menu.

Never do this   Always do this

4. *Stress is a stretch.* It makes you strong or makes you snap.

I am strong.   I am ready to snap.

5. *Exercise is vital to well-being.* Develop a regular program of exercise.

Never do this   Always do this

6. *Rest is the key to recharging.* Put adequate rest in your daily schedule.

Never do this   Always do this

7. *Wellness is an inside-out job.* Make caring for and feeding your soul a priority in your daily plan.

I never consider   Nourishing my soul
food for my soul.   is a priority.

ASK GOD . . .

To give you the vision and desire for a life that is fit, fueled, and free, and to enable you to focus on what to eat (not what to avoid), when to eat, and why you need to eat it.

Day 7

[Read pages 34–36 of *Food For Life.*]

REST, REFLECT, AND REPLENISH

Commit to the Lord whatever you do, and your plans will succeed.

—PROVERBS 16:3

Look over your schedule and circle the unhealthy foods, or ways, that you eat.

REPLENISHING TIP: Spend at least thirty minutes doing something you enjoy (a warm bath, meditating, singing, walking).

WEEKLY ACTION STEP IN REVIEW

Read over your week's diary and circle the suspected problem spots.

What patterns do you see with your eating? _____
_____
_____

What patterns do you see with your exercise (or the lack thereof?) _____
_____
_____

What patterns do you see with your moods and feelings?
_____
_____

Now, read over your answers to the last week's reflection
   questions. Write about the patterns you see, and how you
   feel about the week. _____

_____

_____

In each of the following categories, write down your response
   to this question: *What do I hope to accomplish in the next
   twenty-four days?*

Spiritually: _____

_____

Emotionally: _____

_____

Mentally: _____

_____

Physically: _____

_____

ASK GOD . . .

To fill you with His strength and awesome power.

Week 2

FUELING THE BODY

I, wisdom, dwell together with prudence; I possess knowledge and discretion.
—PROVERBS 8:12

THIS WEEK'S PURPOSE: Living out good intentions

L ife can be super—and super-stressful—all at the same time. We seem to be caught with too much to do and too little time in which to do it. We have never-ceasing, intense demands placed upon us, yet often little supply to meet these demands. Most of us are underfed and underfueled, pushing our bodies through the day without food much like pushing a car up a hill without gasoline. It's not hard to understand why we are overcome with the stresses of life, and why we're more than likely too busy or too tired to do anything about it.

The hope I want to give you is this: We have been created with bodies that will work *for* us and *with* us. To survive, let alone thrive, we need the right foods at the right time in the right balance. I pray that this week will be one in which you will be empowered with the foods that you eat and the knowledge that you are choosing to care for the magnificent body you were created with—and will experience the life you were created for.

ACTION STEP FOR WEEK 2:

Begin a new food diary this week using the "eat right prescription" (eat early, often, balanced, lean, and bright!) as a guide. This is a time to focus on *what to eat* rather than *what to avoid.* Have breakfast every day and power snacks or meals every two-and-one-half to three hours. Each power snack or meal should include a whole complex carbohydrate, lean protein and a brightly colored fruit or vegetable. Also, keep track of the eight to ten glasses of wonderful water you drink each day. (See sample and blank diaries on pages 71–73 of *Food For Life.*) The diary will guide you in choosing nourishing food evenly throughout your day.

VISION STATEMENT

This week you will see eating well as a precious gift you are giving your body—an investment yielding great rewards. As you meet your body's need for the right foods at the right time, you will experience higher, even levels of energy and moods, increased concentration, boosted metabolism and immunities, and an appetite in your control! And as you meet your physical need for proper nourishment, you will be better able to work on the deeper needs of the soul.

Day 8

[Read pages 40–44 of *Food For Life*.]

EAT EARLY, EAT OFTEN

*I rise before dawn and cry for help; I have put my
hope in your word.*

—PSALM 119:147

Here's an important morning formula—start your
day connecting with God, and start yourself with
the right foods; "break the fast" with breakfast! You
don't have a prayer for having stable blood chemistries
or a metabolism burning strong without it. Mom was
right!

If breakfast has been the one meal you usually skip,
why? Check (✔) the breakfast skipping reasons that
apply to you:

- ❏ I skip breakfast to save calories.
- ❏ I don't have time for breakfast.
- ❏ I don't have time to think of myself in the morning.
- ❏ I'm not hungry in the morning.
- ❏ If I eat breakfast, I'm more hungry throughout the
  day.
- ❏ I don't like breakfast foods.

Read pages 46–48 to debunk these myths—it's time to
make the smart investment in breakfast—don't leave
home without it! In your own words, write what benefits you hope to receive from eating breakfast every day:

_____

_____

And, once you get the body burning strong with breakfast, keep it working at peak performance with power snacks smartly planned throughout your day. A strategy of eating smaller, evenly distributed meals undergirds your blood sugars and metabolism with support. This frees you from the constant battle between your appetite and your eating, lack of eating and/or compulsive eating.

Review the power snacks ideas on pages 53–55 of *Food For Life*, and list at least four combos that you are ready to try:

1. _____

2. _____

3. _____

4. _____

List the places you need to keep your power snacks so that they are available to you in your hour of need:

_____

_____

ASK GOD . . .

To help you recognize the way your body was created: to be fueled evenly and often throughout the day. Ask Him to inspire you to get prepared the night before and to wake you up on time. Believe Him to make you sensitive to your body's signals, and trust Him for your appetite to stay in control.

Day 9

[Read pages 45–49 of *Food For Life*.]

EAT BALANCED

Man does not live on bread alone, but on every word that comes from the mouth of God.
—MATTHEW 4:4

Balance is more than just a pretty plate, it's getting the right foods at the right time—including a carbohydrate and protein source at every meal and power snack. Carbohydrates are the perfect energy fuel for your body to burn. The body can also burn protein for energy, but that is not protein's most important function. It has a "higher calling"—being required for boosting the metabolism and immunities, for fluid balance, to build body muscle, and to make beautiful skin, nails, and hair. Protein is the new you!

The healthy goal is to choose carbohydrates in the most whole form possible and thus benefit from both their nutrients and their fiber. This means eating whole grains when you can, such as brown rice, oats, and 100 percent whole grain breads, crackers, cereals, and pastas. Eat whole fruits and vegetables well-washed with skins on, and choose the fruit rather than the fruit juice.

Looking at the listing of simple and complex carbohydrates on pages 61–62 in *Food For Life*, make a list of unfamiliar carbohydrates you would be willing to try.

_____

_____

Add these to your grocery list this week!

Power-building protein is a use-it-or-lose-it nutrient, and high-quality protein foods must be eaten every

23

three to four hours, ideally in the lowest fat form possible. Think more than just meat—include low-fat dairy, soy products, and other beans as protein. Using the "Protein Sources" guide on page 63 of *Food For Life*, list at least five different protein sources you could include in your meal plan.

1. _____   4. _____

2. _____   5. _____

3. _____

Eating well for life is based on this essential balance. Review the recipes beginning on page 93 of *Food For Life* to get an understanding of whole meals giving both carbohydrate and protein.

ASK GOD ...

To help you "break out of the rut" of your past eating habits, and to give you the desire to try new foods. Believe Him for the wisdom to choose foods wisely and in balance.

Day 10

[Read pages 50–57 of *Food For Life*.]

EAT LEAN

This is a lasting ordinance for the generations to come, wherever you live: you must not eat any fat.
—LEVITICUS 3:17

Up-to-date research affirms age-old wisdom and direction: excess fat in our diets is a direct invitation to killer diseases and excess weight. Although we *must* have a certain amount of fat to live well, it is the excess that leads to health risks.

When it comes to health, just knowing fat's negative effects is not enough, you must learn how to reduce the fat in your daily diet. It takes effort and commitment to learn new ways to order healthfully when dining out, to discover positive snack food choices and to trim the excess fat from your grocery selections, and your cooking.

ASK GOD . . .

To empower you to learn new ways to reduce fat, and to give you the wisdom to make wise choices. If you are cooking for a family, believe for the courage and energy to make changes gently, yet definitively.

On the following page you will discover ways to do just that. Check the appropriate box for each suggestion.

The Food Trap

	Need to Do	Doing Now	Will Start
Eat more skinless poultry and fewer red meats. Diminish fat in cooking by grilling, broiling, or roasting on a rack.	___	___	___
Use marinades, flavored vinegars, plain yogurt, or juices when grilling or broiling.	___	___	___
Limit protein portions to five ounces precooked.	___	___	___
Let rice, pasta, potatoes, and vegetables become the centerpiece of your meals.	___	___	___
Use nonstick cooking sprays to brown meats without adding fat. If a recipe calls for basting in butter or meat juices, baste instead with tomato, lemon juice, or stocks.	___	___	___
Skim the fat from soups, stocks, and meat drippings.	___	___	___
Use legumes as a main dish.	___	___	___
Substitute plain, nonfat yogurt or fat-free ricotta cheese in dips or sauces calling for sour cream or mayonnaise.	___	___	___
Use two egg whites or/cup egg substitute in place of one whole egg.	___	___	___
Rarely, if ever, eat animal organ meats, such as liver, sweetbreads, or brains. They are loaded with fats and cholesterol.	___	___	___
Switch from whole-milk dairy products to part-skim or non-fat versions.	___	___	___
Use all-fruit jam on toast in place of butter or margarine.	___	___	___
Order fats on the side when dining out, and use sparingly.	___	___	___
Watch portions.	___	___	___

Day 11

[Read pages 84–88 of *Food For Life.*]

WATER IS THE
BEVERAGE OF CHAMPIONS

*Whoever drinks the water I give him will never
thirst. Indeed the water I give him will become in
him a spring of water welling up to eternal life.*
—JOHN 4:14

The sign by my sink said it all: "Remember: Water is
our most valuable resource." The city of San
Francisco was using the sign to entreat hotel guests
like me to use water wisely and sparingly. I was struck
with the irony that I encourage people to use water
wisely and abundantly. It's God-provided drink to keep
your body working at it's best.

What are the benefits of using water? Check (✔) the
benefits you consider most important to you.

- ❑ Water is an essential nutrient.
- ❑ Water is critical for proper body fluid balance.
- ❑ Water works to release excess stores of fluid. It is *the*
  natural diuretic.
- ❑ Water is the only liquid we consume that doesn't
  require the body to working order to metabolize or
  excrete it.
- ❑ Being a mild laxative, water allows proper bowel
  function and waste elimination.
- ❑ Water is valuable for maintaining proper muscle tone.
- ❑ Water works to keep the skin healthy and resilient.

How much water do we need to drink a day? My

27

answer is always eight to ten glasses per day, and more if you drink coffees, teas, or sodas and when you exercise.

How many glasses of water do you drink daily?

___ 0–3   ___ 4–7   ___ 8 or more

The best replacement fluids for your body when you are dehydrated are water, sparkling water, club soda, and fruit juices. The worst are caffeinated drinks and alcoholic beverages.

The good news: As you begin to properly meet your need by drinking more water, your natural thirst will be restored and so will your well-being!

Check (✔) your major sources of caffeine.

- Coffee
- Tea
- Sodas
- Diet Sodas
- Chocolate
- Decongestants
- Headache remedies
- Stimulants like Vivarin or No-Doze

Can you replace your need for caffeine with the "eat-right prescription" and water?

___Yes   ___I'm willing to try   ___No, not yet

ASK GOD . . .

To refresh you spiritually with His living water and to help you thirst naturally for more of the beverage of champions!

Day 12

[Read pages 89–91 of *Food For Life*.]

VARIETY IS THE SPICE OF LIFE

Blessed are those who hunger and thirst for right-eousness, for they will be filled.
—MATTHEW 5:6

The beautiful thing about good, balanced nutrition is this: Everything fits together in such a perfect way that focusing on eating early, often, balanced, and lean will give you a blessing of essential nutrients. Healthy variety occurs when you make good food choices over a period of time.

The bright coloring of vegetables and fruits is an indication of their nutritional content—the more vivid the color, the more essential nutrients they hold. Check (✔) your favorite ones:

❑ Carrots   ❑ Sweet potatoes
❑ Cantaloupes   ❑ Apricots
❑ Peaches   ❑ Strawberries
❑ Turnips   ❑ Spinach
❑ Broccoli   ❑ Romaine lettuce
❑ Peppers   ❑ Tomatoes
❑ Citrus

Now circle those that you eat on a regular basis, or intend to have more often.

Healthy eating can be enjoyable, tasty, and full of variety. Yet for many people, healthy eating means eating in a rut, a boring rut.

So what's the problem with ruts? Time and time again I see people overindulge as soon as they get the taste of anything more exciting. Then once they get off the track, it becomes very difficult to get back on the track—since, to them, "on track" means returning to the same old, boring rut.

List some of the ways you can bring variety and health to your daily eating plans:

1. _____
2. _____
3. _____
4. _____
5. _____

There are some rut-breaking meal ideas in *Food For Life* on pages 65–70. Try some out in the next few days. Do not let yourself get into a rut and then find yourself overindulging to break the rut.

ASK GOD . . .

To empower you to break out of eating ruts and to enjoy all the healthy ways He has created for you to eat. Thank Him that you are created perfectly, with taste buds to enjoy a rich variety of His foods.

Day 13

[Read pages 119–125 of *Food For Life.*]

FOR THE COOK OF THE HOUSE

Like a city whose walls are broken down is a man who lacks self-control.

—PROVERBS 25:28

The cook of the house needs to break the tasting chain. A cook often eats unconsciously. While cleaning the table, we fight our childhood warnings about wasting food such as: "You need to clean your plate to help the starving children in Asia."

Few people these days have the time or inclination to spend every afternoon preparing the dinner meal. Actually, lack of time can be a major obstacle to a wellness strategy. If your philosophy is, "If it takes longer to cook it than to eat it, forget it!" then the following tips are for you. Underline the time-saving tips you are now implementing and circle the ones you need to start:

▲ When you cook, do so in abundance, then freeze properly portioned leftovers in freezer bags to provide quick meals when you need them.

▲ Keep two empty shoeboxes in your freezer to store ready-made meals. Put main-dish portions in one box, complements (rice, pastas, vegetables) in the other box.

▲ Spend one hour each week preparing some of the basics that will make each night's meal a healthy delight with a minimal effort. For example, cook a big pot of brown rice which can be reheated as needed.

▲ For extra-quick stir-fry, use frozen bags of assorted vegetables.

31

▲ For basic quick salads, tear romaine lettuce and top with tomato, no-oil Italian dressing and a sprinkle of Parmesan.

▲ Keep raw veggies marinating in a no-oil Italian dressing for a quick salad. Add a small can of tuna to make a main dish, and cooked pasta to make a whole meal.

List three tips for avoiding overeating while shopping, cooking, or serving food. Star the ones that will be a particular struggle for you and commit them to prayer.

1. _____
2. _____
3. _____

List two of the time-saving tips that you could employ right away:

1. _____
2. _____

Start your grocery list, adding three to four new items you intend to purchase this week to make your meals and snacks healthier and more appealing. Consult the healthy grocery list on pages 121–123 of *Food For Life.*

1. _____
2. _____
3. _____
4. _____

If you are cooking for a growing family, read the pages about building healthy children once again. Which points strike a chord within you? _____

_____

Remembering that your attitudes about eating are the most significant contribution to your child's eating habits for life, review this list. Write *yes* beside each behavior you exhibit, or *no* beside behaviors you do not exhibit:

___ Binge on food when I'm stressed.
___ I bribe my kids with food (if you're good, you'll get dessert).
___ I punish my kids by denying them food (you can't have dessert, if . . .).
___ I plead with my kids to eat more, or less.
___ I cheer up myself or my kids with food treats (let's go get ice cream!).

If you wrote *yes* by any of these, then the long-term result of your behavior will be that your children learn an improper relationship with food by watching you, and could develop lifelong eating disorders. Instead, we can aspire to teach healthy attitudes about healthy food.

Describe the healthiest food you served your children this week: _____

_____

Remember this: Your children may not always do as you say, but you can be sure they will do as you do.

ASK GOD . . .

To give you the wisdom and motivation to plan ahead with healthy foods for your meals. Believe Him to reveal careless eating, overbuying, and falling into tempting food territory. Ask Him for the strength and wisdom to teach your children healthy messages about food by being their role model.

[Read pages 126–131 of *Food For Life.*]

REST, READ, AND REFLECT

For I know the plans I have for you, declares the Lord.
—JEREMIAH 29:11

REPLENISHING TIP: Spend at least thirty minutes doing something you enjoy (a warm bath, meditating, singing, walking).

WEEKLY ACTION STEP IN REVIEW

Compare your food diaries to the desired guide for your goal (weight loss or maintenance, man or woman) in *Food For Life*, pages 65–70. How did your day-by-day eating differ?

_____

_____

_____

What changes do you want to make for next week?

_____

_____

As you read about stress and its effect on the body, check the following physical reactions that you identify as happening to you:

- ❏ Slowed metabolism
- ❏ Blood sugar fluctuations
- ❏ Bloating/fluid retention
- ❏ Gastric distress
- ❏ Weight gain or weight loss

❑ Fatigue and energy dips
❑ Irritability
❑ Sleep disturbances
❑ Difficulty concentrating
❑ Food cravings
❑ Increased susceptibility to sickness

Put an *x* on the line to indicate the amount of stress you are experiencing right now

_____

None   Light   Moderate   Heavy   Extreme

If you can identify it, list your main source, or sources, of stress at this time:

_____

Although we often can't make the stress in our lives go away, we can learn to respond to stress in a different way. Look up the following scriptures, and jot down what they say to you about your response.

▲ Psalm 37:1, 7 _____
▲ Proverbs 12:25 _____
▲ Matthew 6:25–34 _____
▲ Luke 12:29 _____
▲ 1 Corinthians 7:20–21 _____
▲ Philippians 4:6 _____

ASK GOD . . .

For the strength and vision to take charge of the stress response that you can control—yourself—choosing to keep your body fit and strong. Ask Him to take your worries and anxieties about the things you can't control—situations and people. Receive His peace and health.

NOURISHING THE SOUL

I am the vine; you are the branches. If a man remains in me and I in him, he will bear much fruit; apart from me you can do nothing.

—JOHN 15:5

THIS WEEK'S PURPOSE: To understand that eating well is not enough to keep us well—that wellness is an inside-out job!

As important as it is to identify how life affects us, learning how to diffuse life's stressors is even more critical. To be broken within causes us to feel emotionally, spiritually, and physically drained. Strategic eating, exercise, and rest will enable you to stand strong even when your stress load weighs heavy. It will make all the difference in your being able to "ride the waves" of life rather than drowning in its undertow, because the body is operative from a point of physical strength. However, to get well and stay well, it is also critical to meet our deeper needs—to feed our souls with the right kind of soul food.

This means making peace with food, with our bodies, with our feelings, with God, and with others.

ACTION STEP FOR WEEK 3:

Choose foods and portions for your meals and snacks based on the desired guide on pages 65–70 of *Food For Life*. Keep in mind that these are guides for minimum portions and proper balance to achieve your desired goals for healthy living. Get started with these amounts for the next two weeks to allow your body to stabilize before making adjustments, and keep a diary of what you eat and drink, when and how much, along with exercise times and types.

If you haven't already begun to experiment with the meal ideas and recipes on pages 92–118, it's time to break out of the rut! Select at least three recipes you intend to try this week.

Daily review your diary to see where you've gotten off track, looking for the impact of stress and changes in routine. Circle in red the third and fifth day and pay close attention to desires to "go back" to old ways.

VISION STATEMENT

This week will illuminate the truth of how we were made, our optimal operating design, to know who we are, and whose we are. At the end of the third week, new healthy habits have been established.

Day 15

[Read pages 133–135 of *Food For Life*.]

BUILD THE STRESS-FIGHTING WEAPONS ARSENAL

For the weapons of our warfare are not carnal, but mighty through God to the pulling down of strongholds.

—2 CORINTHIANS 10:4, KJV

Properly timed and balanced eating can keep your energy level high and your body actively metabolizing the nutrients you eat, working on a deflective shield for the body. In addition, balanced eating energizes you for exercise and allows for more restful sleep, both of which serve as swords to cut away stress. We need to employ all of these weapons to offset the negative symptoms of stress—we need a *sword* and a *shield*.

Below is a list of different kinds of exercise. Prioritize your three favorite types of exercise and circle those you do, or could do, regularly each week.

___ Walking
___ Running or jogging
___ Aerobic dancing or stepping
___ Bike riding
___ Swimming
___ Working out on weight equipment
___ Playing sports
___ Other: _____

Discover the body's need for exercise beyond weight

38

issues. Exercise is an offensive weapon in the war against stress. It's a stress-buster.

Incredibly, only one activity other than exercise produces stress-busting endorphins: laughter. When you laugh you are telling your body that the stressful circumstance is no big deal! It can't be bad if you laugh, so lighten up and laugh. Read Proverbs 14:30, and write it down in your own words:

_____

_____

The next time the enemy of life attempts a strike at you and tries to stress you out, pick up your sharpened sword and laugh in his face.

ASK GOD ...

To give you His perspective on stress: There's no reason for stress to paralyze us in its grip. We are victors, not victims. Ask Him to motivate you to exercise and to fill you with joy and laughter.

Day 16

[Read pages 136–144 of *Food For Life.*]

EXERCISE FOR THE DISCIPLINED SOUL

The Lord delights in the way of the man whose steps he has made firm; although he stumble, he will not fall, for the Lord upholds him with his hand.
—PSALM 37:23

Proper nutrition without exercise is like a car without tires—the body may look good, but it won't go anywhere. Exercise is the offensive tool to cut off the body's stress response. As many as 80 percent of those who start an exercise routine drop out soon after starting, and of the 40 percent of Americans who exercise, only 20 percent reap any aerobic benefits. We need help in staying committed to exercise.

Exercise:
▲ increases metabolism and decreases appetite.
▲ increases your protection against disease.
▲ breaks the plateaus of weight loss.
▲ is nature's best tranquilizer.
▲ is a vital factor in promoting excellent bone growth and maintenance.

Here is an exercise guide to being F.I.T.T. After each point, complete the sentence:

Frequency: 4–6 days a week.
I exercise ____ days a week.

Intensity: At a level where you feel slightly out of breath without gasping.
I exercise by _____.

40

Time: 30–60 minutes at a time of day when you feel good and your schedule allows a routine to be built.

The time of day I feel good about exercising is_____.

Type: The best workout works all the muscles of your body. Include warmup, cool down, conditioning, and aerobic exercise.

My favorite form of regular exercise is _____

For those of us who do not like any type of exercise, I suggest fitness walking. Try walking a mile a day. Check how long it took you to walk that mile. Increase your pace so that you can walk two miles in thirty minutes and then three miles in forty-five minutes. Plan on getting some walking in every day or at least four days a week.

Know yourself and how not to push yourself over your abilities. Start slowly and avoid overtaxing yourself. Let exercise be something you choose to do for life.

What three motivational factors would help you to choose exercise as a way of life?
1. _____
2. _____
3. _____

ASK GOD . . .

To give you a new perspective about exercise and to inspire and strengthen you in your commitment to a daily exercise routine. Believe Him to make "your steps firm" and to uphold you with His hand.

[Read pages 145–151 of *Food For Life.*]

REVITALIZING REST

It still remains that some will enter that rest.

—HEBREWS 4:6

To enjoy life spiritually, emotionally, relationally, and physically, we must be recharged and renewed during times of rest. You may protest, "Recharge and rest—ha! You don't know my life. You don't understand the demands on me."

Allowing ourselves to be robbed of restful sleep cheats us of half our mental powers to carry us through the next day.

Even Jesus required quiet time to maintain His peace. Read Luke 5:15–16, and study how Jesus got some rest and quiet time.

Those who do not get proper rest can burn out, get sick, and sometimes become bitter. There are danger signs that we are not getting enough rest and sleep. Check (✔) any that you are presently experiencing:

❑ Grouchiness   ❑ Forgetfulness
❑ Indecisiveness   ❑ Lack of humor
❑ Lack of creativity   ❑ Lack of
❑ Irritableness   spontaneity
❑ Other: _____

Making rest a lifestyle is choosing to give our cares to God in our waking hours as well as in our sleeping hours. We enter rest when we let go of all we don't want, won't use, and don't need. We feel uplifted and drawn to new challenges because we aren't struggling to carry the old. Here are some tips to keep your body keyed for restful sleep. Circle the tips you need the most:

▲ Exercise and keep fit.
▲ Be clock-driven. Block sleep as part of your schedule.
▲ Choose nighttime snacks wisely.
▲ Minimize noise when you sleep.
▲ Rest more during the day.

You also need time for time-outs during the day. These may be 15–30 minute breaks or longer in which you rest, exercise, meditate on God's Word, pray, and spend quiet time with the Lord. Describe when your time-outs take place during the day.
My quiet times are _____.

ASK GOD . . .

To help you carve out time for rest and replenishment and to show you the truth about quiet times—that they are His time with you to allow you to see your worries as He does: small stuff that belongs to Him.

[Read pages 152–159 of *Food For Life.*]

WELLNESS IS AN INSIDE-OUT JOB

I praise you because I am fearfully and wonderfully made; your works are wonderful, I know that full well.

—PSALM 139:14

Eating well is not enough to make us well. More than caring for and feeding our physical bodies, living well means caring for and feeding our souls. We must feast on God's truth.

The truth is God values us highly. Read Psalm 139 and jot down at least five ways that God shows His care for us:

1. _____

2. _____

3. _____

4. _____

5. _____

As you start taking care of yourself and nourishing your physical body, new feelings may bubble to the surface. These feelings need to be processed in new, healthy ways to prevent them from becoming logjams to your wellness.

Remember that emotions produce energy. If we don't release that energy, we must work to keep it in. Keeping emotional energy buried can result in a big bang that expresses itself destructively in our physical beings and in our relationships.

Are you aware of "suppressed" or "unprocessed" feelings affecting your eating habits or health?

__ no __ somewhat __ sometimes ___yes ___intensely

Here are some ways to release repressed emotional energy. Underline those you could utilize:

▲ Allow yourself to feel your feelings.
▲ Write in a journal.
▲ Lift up how you feel to God in prayer.
▲ Spend time in God's Word.
▲ Sing praises and prayers.
▲ Create something with your hands.
▲ Walk.
▲ Share with trusted friends.

Denial is an addictive tool for survival but a destructive coping device that destroys ourselves and others. With God's help, meet your feelings face-to-face. Bringing them out into the open and letting them go will renew your mind and release you to experience God's healing and joy.

ASK GOD . . .

To help you face and release your feelings.

[Read pages 162–168 of *Food For Life.*]

THE CHALLENGE OF CHANGE

See, I am doing a new thing! Now it springs up; do you not perceive it?

—ISAIAH 43:19

Change is part of your life, and it is one of your greatest challenges. The first and biggest step in the challenge of change is to recognize the need for change and passionately desire to bring it about.

Desire to change is critical, since change is hard to face and even harder to effect in our lives. It stirs up old fears and can be terrifying. We can remain stuck in old patterns simply because of fear. If we feel stressed and out of control, or paralyzed by fear, we are afraid to change.

There are five difficult stages we must go through in order to embrace fully any change in our lives. On the line next to each one, indicate where you are right now.

▲ Fear of the unknown _____

▲ Fear of failure _____

▲ Fear of commitment _____

▲ Fear of disapproval _____

▲ Fear of success _____

How do we overcome fear? We can take the following steps:

1. Admit fear—look it in the face.

2. Work hard—take classes, talk to others, and learn how to overcome fear.
3. Make a tough decision—decide to move beyond the fear.
4. Be ready for pain—go through the pain associated with overcoming fear.
5. Experience joy and transformation—accept change.

Complete these sentences:

▲ My greatest fear right now is _____.

▲ The stage I'm going through to overcome this fear is _____

_____.

▲ The next step I need to take in overcoming this fear is_____

_____.

What is the major change you were trying to accomplish when you began this guide?_____

_____

What changes do you now expect?_____

_____

ASK GOD . . .

To deliver you from fear of change into a spirit of love, power, and a strong mind.

47

[Read pages 169–182 of *Food For Life*.]

OVERCOMING SETBACKS AND SABOTAGE

We must pay more careful attention, therefore, to what we have heard, so that we do not drift away.
—HEBREWS 2:1

Even after you have adjusted physically to a new way of eating and looking at food, you will sometimes crave foods you used to love. You will walk through vulnerable times that tempt you to eat unhealthily. Check (✔) the most vulnerable times for you:

- ❏ Parties
- ❏ Stressful events
- ❏ Social events where food is the main attraction
- ❏ Going out to eat
- ❏ Watching someone eat something unhealthy that you used to love
- ❏ Traditional holiday meals
- ❏ Fatigue
- ❏ Other: _____

It will take at least five to six days before your new healthy eating begins to feel comfortable physically.

I will describe for you what most people experience. Write down your experience and feelings for that day(s).

Days 1 and 2: Most people feel slightly sluggish, irritable, and dissatisfied with their eating habits.
I feel _____.

Day 3: This is one of the difficult days. The body begins to feel the chemical change and cries out for food. This day is a struggle, but not impossible to overcome.

I feel _____.

Day 4: This day will not be so difficult.

I feel _____.

Day 5: This is the day of the ravenous appetite. Expect to be hungry for food. Many eat a meal and still think: *What else is there to eat?*

I feel _____.

Days 6 and 7: By now it is getting easier. Most people have more energy and self-control.

I feel _____.

When you fall, just get up, forgive yourself, and go back to living healthy. Eating well is a lot like learning to ride a bike. No matter how often you fall, don't lose heart. The more often you try, the better you will get at it. Once you've learned to eat healthy, you will never want to return to unhealthy eating habits.

Look at your diary for the last six days. Did you experience the feelings explained on pages 169–170, particularly on days three and five?

___yes ___somewhat ___I didn't pay attention ___No

Once you experience how good it feels to eat and live healthy, you will be more more aware, and intolerant, of feeling bad and tired.

Another major challenge to personal change will be dealing with the reactions of friends and family. Your change may be as scary to them as it is to you. They are losing a familiar you and getting to know a new you.

They may have liked the old you a little better, particularly if the old you met their needs—even at the expense of your own.

The best way to respond to sabotage even from friends and family is, "Just say no!" Who are the hardest people to say no to when they knowingly or unknowingly sabotage your healthy lifestyle? Prioritize from the most difficult (1), to the least difficult (6).

___ Family
___ Friends
___ Work associates
___ Sports associates
___ Community or church people at an event
___ Other: _____

Write this in your own words, personalized, on a 3x5 card and refer to it often: *"The only person capable of gaining the freedom you desire for yourself is you. Another person may not force you to change or prevent you from doing so. Another person's words and actions may have an effect on you, but ultimately it is you who decides your actions.*

Practice saying this: *"I don't care for any, thank you."*
Never say: *"I can't eat that."*

ASK GOD . . .

To alert you to and navigate you through temptation and the actions of misguided people, and to keep your foot from the deadly snare.

[Read pages 177–178 of *Food For Life*.]

REST, REFLECT, AND REORDER

*Turn my eyes away from worthless things; renew
my life according to your word.*

—PSALM 119:37

REPLENISHING TIP: Spend at least thirty minutes doing
something you enjoy: a warm bath, meditating, singing,
or walking.

READING AND REFLECTION

A particular agent of sabotage to our renewing of the
mind is the scale. This is especially true for the reformed
dieter—the one who has finally accepted that health and
fitness is based on caring for the body. The scale has no
indicator that shows how much of your weight is muscle
mass, water weight, or fat. It just shows a number.

Yet for years, the scale has been used as a "god" to tell
us if we've been good or bad, if we should be happy or
sad, if we can eat—or have to starve—on any given day.

Check the statements that express your attitude
towards the scale:

___ If I'm going to give up everything I enjoy in life (my
favorite foods), I surely better get a payoff! If the scale
doesn't budge, I yell, "Not fair! If I'm not going to
lose, I might as well be eating."
___ If the scale shows a weight loss, I celebrate how
"good" I've been, and, of course, celebrate with food.
___ If I lose five pounds, I'm sure it's fat.
___ If I gain five pounds, I think it might be fluid.

___ I weigh every morning, or sometimes three times a day to see if I'm gaining weight from the food I'm eating.

___ The scale seems to have a magnetic power that pulls me towards it.

Could you weigh yourself right now, then not weigh yourself again for a month? Could you trust in the healthy way you are choosing to eat; trust in how you feel your body is responding, and not in what the scale is reading? Can you trust in God to direct your eating rather than the scale god?

Giving up your reliance on the scale can be more difficult than giving up overeating. But give it a try, it will be a major step in breaking out of the diet mentality—and a major step in your walk of freedom!

WEEKLY ACTION STEP IN REVIEW

Review your food diaries in the light of what you have learned in these three weeks. Compared to your first week, what changes have you made in your eating and exercise patterns?

_____

_____

Compared to your first week, what changes do you see in terms of energy, mood, concentration, appetite control, and your overall sense of well-being?

_____

_____

What areas of your eating and exercise need more focus to improve? _____

_____

What new things are you doing to nourish your soul?

ASK GOD . . .

To fill you with His grace for change, to enable you to stay on course, and to stay a champion. Thank Him, rejoice with Him in the changes in your perspective about yourself, your choices, and your relationship with Him.

Breaking Free and Staying Free From the Food Trap

My eyes are ever on the Lord, for only He will release my feet from the snare.

—Psalm 25:15

This Week's Purpose: To embrace healthy beliefs and be set free from the food trap, or any trap, of life.

A healthy relationship with food regards food as the nourishment God created it to be. There is no good or bad food, no legal or cheat food. Food is simply food. Our attitude toward food can make all the difference in whether or not we will have a healthy lifestyle.

Food is a trap when it is used as a substitute for love, friendship, or success, or when it's used to cover up more serious emotional issues. Unhealthy eating or overeating can become a way of coping with life.

Weekly Action Step in Review

If you've not yet begun to keep a journal, now is the time to begin. Revisit pages 156–159 in *Food For Life* to guide you into this miraculous journey to a new kind of freedom. If journaling is new for you, be patient with yourself. You may not be used to feeling feelings, let alone recording them. You may find that just reviewing yesterday's writings in this guidebook, and writing about how that makes you feel, will be a good place to start.

VISION STATEMENT

By looking clearly at the emotional you and your relationship between food and your body, you can name the problem, and begin the process of healing—you can see the hidden controls in life be broken. New relationships with God, yourself, and others can meet your spiritual and emotional needs. Food no longer needs to be the protective barrier between you and the world, or between you and God.

[Read pages 179–181 of *Food For Life*.]

SABOTAGED BY SHAME?

Search me, O God, and know my heart; test me and know my anxious thoughts. See if there is any offensive way in me, and lead in the way everlasting.

—PSALM 139:23–24

"I know the enemy, and he is me." Self-sabotage is fueled by fear and shame. Do any of these statements strike a cord of familiarity about how you feel about yourself?

__ I don't make mistakes, I am a mistake.
__ God was on a coffee break when I was being created.
__ I'm different, less valuable, than other people.
__ I can't do anything right.
__ I'll never get this weight off.
__ If only I was better, I could _____.
__ If only I was thinner, I could _____.

If you checked one or more of these statements, you may be operating from a sense of shame, one of the most powerful sabotage agents for healthy change. If you believe you are junk, why wouldn't you want to treat yourself like junk and feed yourself junk food?

You can overcome the self-sabotage of shame from words that you speak destructively about yourself, from abandonment that has been caused by others, and from emotional or physical abuse. You do not have to cover past shame with food. Read 1 John 1 and Romans 5, and then summarize in your own words:

What God has done with my shame is:

_____
_____
_____
_____

Ask God . . .

To forgive you of your past and release you from shame, to help you forgive others for hurts they have inflicted on you through words, actions, or abuse. Believe Him for the strength to forgive yourself.

[Read pages 181–189 of *Food For Life.*]

STUCK IN THE FOOD TRAP?

Be careful, or your hearts will be weighed down with . . . the anxieties of life, and that day will close on you unexpectedly like a trap.

—LUKE 21:34

For some, food is a source of pleasure. For others, it is a response to an emotion. Such response can become a great danger—millions of Americans are emotionally dependent on food.

Put yourself to the test. What do you eat when you feel certain emotions? Complete each sentence if it applies to you:

▲ When happy, I like to eat _____.
▲ When depressed, I like to eat _____.
▲ When stressed, I like to eat _____.
▲ When relaxing, I like to eat _____.
▲ When frustrated, I like to eat _____.

If you completed any of the above sentences, you connect certain foods to certain emotions. That may lead you to the food trap.

Scripture is full of illustrations about food and gluttony, messages often ignored. Food and finances are two vulnerable issues for us because we can't live without them. So, we must apply the spiritual fruit of self-control to these issues (Gal. 5:22–23). Using food for immediate self-gratification makes food a false god.

We all desire change in our lives. If you are in a food

trap, identifying the problem is the first step on the road to freedom and change.

ASK GOD . . .

To set you free from the food trap and to use food as it was created—a source of nourishment for our bodies.

[Read pages 190–193 of *Food For Life*.]

IS THE REFRIGERATOR LIGHT THE LIGHT OF YOUR LIFE?

Jesus . . . said, "I am the light of the world. Whoever follows me will never walk in darkness, but will have the light of life."

—JOHN 8:12

We use food for purposes it was never meant to fulfill. Look at the unhealthy and false beliefs listed below. Indicate your present beliefs about each one with an *x*.

1. Food (or dieting) helps me cope with stress, frustration, and the insecurities of life.

_____

Strongly believe   Don't believe

2. Food (or dieting) fills the gaps in my life. Food can be a friend and companion who is with me no matter what.

_____

Strongly believe   Don't believe

3. Food (or dieting) gives me a sense of identity and control. Loving and controlling food are a lot safer than loving people.

_____

Strongly believe   Don't believe

4. Food (or dieting) helps me sabotage the "perfect image." If I am an obedient, people-pleasing person, I can use food as a nice way to be bad.

Strongly believe   Don't believe

5. Food (or dieting) helps me deal with deep-seated emotions and feelings. Keeping my mind on food can keep it off the issues of my heart.

Strongly believe   Don't believe

If you strongly believe any of these statements, then you are growing unhealthy attitudes about food. The satisfied feeling we get from food fills the gaps only temporarily. Typically, the more we eat the more depressed we get.

ASK GOD . . .

To help you see food as it was created. To meet your physical needs in a pleasurable way, but never to be "the light of your life." Ask Him to fill you with His light that shines in the dark areas of your life. Believe Him for the wisdom and strength to identify and deal with the real issues of life in healthy ways, not with food or any other unhealthy substitute.

[Read pages 194–199 of *Food For Life*.]

LOOKING BACK

*But one thing I do: Forgetting what is behind and
straining toward what is ahead, I press on.*

—PHILIPPIANS 3:13

As adults we may appear to be coping with day-to-day life. But all the while, the child in us may be suffering from an overwhelming sense of shame, guilt, self-denial, distrust, or responsibility—that is, taking on burdens that are not ours to carry.

We have all developed faulty systems for coping in one way or another. It is part of humanity. It is based on the same lies used on Eve in the garden (Gen. 3:1–3):

1. No one, not even God, can or will meet your needs.

2. If you are going to get your needs met, you'd better develop your own system for getting them met.

3. If you get your needs met in an unhealthy way or, as Adam and Eve did, in a sinful way, you won't experience any negative consequences.

If you believe any of these lies and did not learn as a child how to meet your emotional and spiritual needs properly, you will, as an adult, be more susceptible to life's traps—including the food trap.

Most of us learned our food attitudes, as well as other

attitudes, from our families. In a healthy family, where personal thoughts and feelings are listened to and given value, a child has the opportunity to develop a sense of identity and self-esteem. But not all of us were raised in such healthy families.

As a result, food may become an escape or trap.

Eating dependencies most often come out of three types of unhealthy family systems. Read *Food For Life* for full details (page 197).

Put an *x* on the line that defines your family as you were growing up:

_____

Healthy   Not sure   Unhealthy

Which of these family systems do you suspect you may have grown-up in:

    ❏ basically healthy   ❏ perfectionistic
    ❏ chaotic   ❏ overprotective

ASK GOD . . .

To set you free from any unhealthy family patterns of the past. If appropriate, praise God for being raised in a healthy family.

[Read pages 200–203 of *Food For Life.*]

LOOKING BACK
WITH UNDERSTANDING

All this is from God, who reconciled us to himself through Christ and gave us the ministry of reconciliation.

—2 CORINTHIANS 5:18

What systems are making you powerless to break free of the food trap? Allow any new information that surfaces as you complete these lessons to be transformed by the renewing of your mind (Rom. 12:1–2).

In the space provided below, answer the following questions for yourself.

1. Look at the relationships in your family—between your mother and father, grandmother and grandfather, parent and children, sibling and sibling. What dynamics characterized each relationship?

_____

_____

2. What strengths did you learn from the family systems? From your mother? From your father?

_____

_____

3. What weaknesses or negative character traits did you learn?

_____

_____

4. What did your family teach you about God?

_____

_____

Based on these thoughts, identify present-day eating problems you may have as a result of your childhood upbringing:

Do you feel as though you have struggled with bulimic or anorexic symptoms? _____

_____

You may need professional help to overcome these treacherous traps. If so, go for help. You *are* worth helping, and you deserve to live well!

Write a prayer forgiving yourself and your family for past unhealthy attitudes and behaviors:

_____

_____

_____

ASK GOD ...

To save you and set you free from all the world's traps—including the food trap. Give Him praise for His Son Jesus Christ who sets us free.

Day 27

[Read pages 204–208 of *Food For Life*.]

RELEASING THE PAST

Therefore, if any man be in Christ, he is a new crea-
ture: old things are passed away; behold, all things
are become new.
                                    —2 CORINTHIANS 5:17, KJV

Attempt to put into words the eating problem you feel you may have:

_____

_____

Who is a trustworthy person whom you can share this problem with, and pray with?

_____

_____

Two major problems prevent us from being renewed and restored: Not forgiving, and not receiving forgiveness. Difficult as it may be, it is nonetheless within our will to choose forgiveness, and it is God's awesome power and grace that brings it to be.

If you were to write a letter such as the one on page 207 of *Food For Life*, to whom would you write?

_____

_____

If you chose to write such a letter, describe how you felt after you wrote it, and lifted it up to God:

_____

_____

66

Write about this in your journal.

Read Genesis 50. You can never go back and relive your early life, but as Joseph proclaimed in Genesis 50:20, God can restore what has been robbed from you and use for good what may have been meant for evil.

ASK GOD ...

To help you see the past just as it is, the past. Ask Him to give you the strength and momentum to take your eyes off the problem, or its cause, and to focus on a life filled with freedom, peace, and joy.

[Read pages 209–210 of *Food For Life.*]

REFLECTION, REPLENISHMENT, AND REST

Now to him who is able to do immeasurably more than all we ask or imagine, according to his power that is at work within us.

—EPHESIANS 3:20

We are not born free—we are born to be free. Spiritual freedom comes with knowing God and His desires for our lives. He desires for us to live in His power. The same power that raised Jesus from the dead gives us victory over our past, over our shame, over the traps of life. His power is ours when we accept His redeeming grace and ask His Spirit to live within us.

God is not just a higher power that I'm reaching up to. God in His love has reached down to us; He empowers us by living within us.

What do you need to do? Submit your body, soul, and spirit to God, and receive the gift of His love and power.

ASK GOD . . .

To come into your life—and your problems—with His power and strength. Ask Him to rule over every area of your life, including the area of eating and food dependency. Believe Him for victory and freedom—day by day, hour by hour, meal by meal, choice after choice. Ask Him to write 3 John 1:2 on your heart, making it clear to you that His desire for you is for you to prosper and be in health.

[Read pages 212–213 of *Food For Life.*]

LIVING HEALTHY AND FREE

But thanks be to God! He gives us the victory [making us more than conquerors] through our Lord Jesus Christ.
— 1 CORINTHIANS 15:57

Acknowledging that "yesterday ended last night," and that you have completed reading the book *Food For Life*, define your own personal plan for eating for life, including at least three key steps or activities you have committed to—for life.

_____

_____

_____

Remember these vital keys to living healthy and free:

▲ *Prayer*
_____ In my new way of living, I commit to pray every day.

▲ *Being guided by the Holy Spirit*
_____ In my new way of living, I commit to enjoy daily quiet time and meditation to hear and be directed by the Holy Spirit.

▲ *Choosing to eat well of the food that gives life*
_____ In my new way of living, I commit to daily choose to eat to thrive.

▲ *Staying in accountable relationships*

____ In my new way of living, I commit to daily contact with people who are special to me and supportive of me.

▲ *Staying committed and finishing strong*

____ In my new way of living, I commit to live in freedom every day.

If this is your vision, then catch the freedom in Christ to live and eat healthy. Don't let any life trap hinder you another minute! If you will commit to these keys, sign your name on the line below:

_____
(signed)

_____
(date)

Day 30

[Read pages 211–213 in *Food For Life*.]

A Food-For-Life Vision

This I recall to my mind, therefore have I hope. It is of the Lord's mercies that we are not consumed, because His compassions fail not. They are new every morning: great is thy faithfulness.
— LAMENTATIONS 3:21–23, KJV

Congratulations! You've done what few people do—you've followed through on a vision and a commitment. Research tells us that these thirty days have worked to seal your behavior changes related to your eating, exercise, and rest into lifetime patterns. Certainly by now you are noticing real changes in your thinking patterns as well. Your health and your appearance may be reflecting these changes.

But these thirty days have really become the beginning of your new life of wellness—as you continue on the positive path you have set your eyes upon. To finish the race before you, perseverance and faithfulness will be required. You will need to continue to put into practice what you now believe. To believe is to follow.

You've spent the last thirty days ending each session with "Asking God." Use this day to tell God "Thank You" for the wondrous works He has done, for the awesome power of His name, for the power of His grace. My prayer is that you will—through His help and by His power—overcome every obstacle in the way of living in freedom every day!

God, I thank You for _____

_____

_____

_____

In Your name, Amen!

Leader's Guide

This devotional study is an excellent resource for group study, including such settings as:

▲ Sunday school and other church classes
▲ Prayer groups
▲ Bible study groups
▲ Small group ministries, home groups, and accountability groups
▲ Study groups for youth and adults

Before the first session:

1. Inform everyone interested or already participating in the group about the meeting time, date, and place.
2. Make certain that everyone has a copy of this devotional study guide and a copy of *Food For Life*.
3. Ask group members to begin their daily encounters using this guide. While each session will not strictly adhere to a seven-day schedule, group members who faithfully do a devotional each day will be prepared to share in the group sessions.
4. Pray for the Holy Spirit to guide, teach, and help each participant.
5. Be certain that the place where you meet has a chalkboard, white board, or flip chart with appropriate writing materials. It is also best to meet in a setting with movable—not fixed—seating.

LIVING WELL

1. Welcome group members as they arrive.
2. Open with prayer, asking God for the desire and motivation to eat right. Read Philippians 4:13 aloud.
3. Open a general group discussion with the question: "How is the *Food For Life* approach to eating different than most diet plans you know about?"
4. List these differences on a chalkboard or flip chart.
5. Divide into pairs; allow each pair to share their responses to the questions in Day 1.
6. As a group, have people share how many diet plans they have been on in the past five years. Have fun with this.
7. Ask several people to read the scriptures from Day 2. Discuss what the Bible has to say about our thought lives.
8. In pairs, share responses to the questions in Day 3, and the food traps discovered on Day 4.
9. Go around the group and ask each person to share two of the completed sentences from Day 5 that they feel comfortable in sharing. As a group, discuss: "How can we best get our bodies working for and with us?"
10. In pairs, have group members share their responses to the Seven Secrets for Staying

Fit, Fueled, and Free, from Day 6.

11. As a group, share how people feel about eating early in the day. Identify the "morning people" and "night people." Ask how that affects eating habits.

12. In pairs, invite each member to share one goal he or she has for the course and to pray with one another for that goal. Then close in prayer.

Session 2

EATING WELL

1. Welcome all the group members as they arrive and ask them to sit with the partner they had last time. Begin the session in prayer.

2. Read Romans 8:21 aloud, and ask people to share how that verse fits their lives in respect to eating healthy food.

3. As a total group, get responses to this statement: *I grab snacks when* _____.

4. Go around the group asking people to share their responses from Day 8–10 about eating early, eating often, eating balanced, and eating lean.

5. Ask people to share favorite breakfast foods, and to describe the breakfast hour.

6. Discuss favorite healthy snack foods.

7. Discuss these questions: "What does Pam Smith mean by eating balanced? What keeps you from eating balanced?"

8. Discuss the best ways various people have found for eating lean.

9. In pairs, share their attitudes about eating from Day 13, and discuss how they can be avoided.

10. As a group, discuss the number of glasses of water each person drinks a day. Then have fun toasting each other with a glass of water and saying, "Drink eight of these for health!"

11. Close the group in a circle of prayer. Ask each person to pray silently that the person on each side will eat early, eat often, eat balanced, and eat lean.

12. Close with sentence prayers for the whole group, asking God to inspire each person to put into action what they have learned.

IT IS WELL WITH MY SOUL

1. Welcome the group as they arrive, and read Proverbs 12:25 aloud. Discuss how depression and stress can tempt us to overeat or to eat unhealthy foods.

2. As a group, discuss ways to put variety into our eating plans.

3. Discuss ways people have found to help children learn how to eat healthy. List those ways on a chalkboard or flip chart.

4. In pairs, share how each person was raised as a child to think about food. Was food used to punish, reward, or handle emotions in their home as a child?

5. From Day 16, discuss the exercise guide to being F.I.T.T. Allow each group member to share.

6. On the chalkboard or flip chart, list all the comfort foods that the group enjoys.

7. In pairs, share how each person will now handle stress by eating healthy, exercising, getting rest, and drinking plenty of water.

8. Ask everyone in the group to share how they rest, relax, laugh, and deal with fatigue.

9. Read Luke 5:15–16, and discuss how Jesus got some rest and quiet time.

10. Go around the group and invite each person to respond to this statement: "The next step I need to take toward living a healthy life is

_____."

11. Form a circle and invite each person to pray a sentence prayer: "God, I ask You to help me _____."

12. Close the session with a prayer from the leader, thanking God for rest, exercise, and healthy foods.

Session 4

BREAK FREE, LIVE FREE

1. Welcome everyone as they arrive. Read
    Isaiah 43:19 aloud. Discuss the new things
    God has been doing in individual lives
    during this study.

2. Discuss the unhealthy and false beliefs you
    studied in Day 24. Pause to ask God to help
    each group member overcome these beliefs.

3. In pairs, share the present-day eating prob-
    lems that group members may have as a
    result of their childhood upbringing.

4. In pairs, ask partners to share the hardest
    thing they have had to do or change during
    this study.

5. As a group, list on a chalkboard or flip chart
    all the healthy attitudes and action steps
    individuals can remember from his or her
    personal study.

6. Ask each person in the group to respond to
    each of the following statements:

▲   The most important thing I learned in this study is

_____.

▲ My greatest fear about continuing to live healthy is

_____.

▲ One strength I have discovered in myself is

_____.

7. In pairs, invite the partners to pray for one another to face their fears and temptations and to overcome them.

8. As a group, allow individuals to share responses to the following statements:

▲ The biggest change in my life during this study is

_____.

▲ My vision for myself in the future is

_____.

9. Close the group in a prayer circle. Invite each person to thank God for what they have discovered about healthy eating and living through this study.

OTHER BOOKS AND TAPES

BY PAMELA M. SMITH, R.D.

EAT WELL—LIVE WELL

The nutrition guide and cookbook for healthy, productive people. A bestseller, this large, hardback edition presents "The Ten Commandments of Great Nutrition" in detail, along with cooking tips, menu planning, grocery shopping, a dining-out guide and a large cookbook section of innovative recipes that can be prepared in a time-saving manner. Meal plans are also included.

THE GOOD LIFE: A HEALTHY COOKBOOK

A wonderful feast of Pam's most savory recipes. This cookbook offers complete meals for breakfast, lunch, and dinner, plus scrumptious desserts and power snack ideas. For the novice or gourmet cook, this book is designed for everyone to enjoy—and it's beautiful too!

"LIVE THE GOOD LIFE" GUIDEBOOK

A six-week plan for embracing your new life of wellness—a life with good food and good health!

PERFECTLY PREGNANT

This is the expectant mother's handbook. Latest information on how to nourish mother and baby properly. Included is a wonderful, proven solution for morning sickness. Handwritten. Tasty recipes too. Meal plans are included.

THE SEVEN SECRETS TO
LIVING THE GOOD LIFE

In this dynamic four-tape series, you will learn how to fit healthy living into your busy schedule, turbo-charge your metabolism and immune system, seal the "energy leaks" in your body and recharge and refuel while you lean down. Pam demonstrates her healthy and delicious cooking techniques and gives easy tips for traveling and dining out healthfully. This four-part series is available in audio and video.

THE FOOD TRAP SEMINAR

On this audiotape album, hear Pamela Smith present a live seminar covering the physical, emotional, and spiritual needs that we have and how to meet and nourish these needs properly. A nutritional strategy for dealing with stress is also presented. Very practical and informative.

ALIVE AND WELL IN THE FAST LANE

A lighthearted and informative nutritional guidebook for the whole family—in a fun, handwritten, and illustrated format. Includes tips for healthy eating on the run.

For more information on books,
tapes and seminars, please write or call:

PAMELA M. SMITH, R.D.
P. O. Box 541009
Orlando, FL 32854
800.896.4010 (orders)
407.855.8630 (information)

To order *Food For Life, Eat Well—Live Well,*
The Good Life: A Healthy Cookbook, or to book
a Food Trap Seminar in your church, contact:

CREATION HOUSE
600 Rinehart Road
Lake Mary, FL 32746
800.283.8494
Fax: 800.283.4561

About the Author

PAMELA M. SMITH is a nationally known nutritionist, best-selling author and culinary consultant. She has been featured on "The Today Show," CNN News, "The 700 Club," "Focus on the Family" and a number of other nationally broadcast radio talk shows.

Pamela is the founder of Nutritional Counseling Services in Orlando, Florida, one of the original private practices of dietetics in America. She is the nutritionist for the Orlando Magic NBA team and for other professional athletes nationwide. She has also served as consultant to industry giants such as Walt Disney World and Hyatt Hotels and Resorts and is the director of culinary development for General Mills Restaurants, New Business Division.

Pamela counsels her clients on an interactive basis, helping them to identify and alter eating and behavioral habits for disease prevention; peak performance in sports; child and family nutrition; weight loss; dining-out strategies; and, very important, stress and emotional implications.

Her books include *Eat Well—Live Well,* a best-selling nutrition guide and cookbook; *Perfectly Pregnant,* a nutrition book for the expectant mother; *The Good Life,* and *Food for Life,* an in-depth look at the physical, emotional and spiritual aspects of nourishing our bodies.

She received her degree in nutrition from Florida State University and completed her American Dietetic Association internship at Miami-Valley Hospital in Dayton, Ohio. She has completed continuing education at the Cooper Clinic in Dallas, Texas, as well as through the Harvard Medical School. She was also the nutrition instructor at the University of Central Florida, Department of Nursing.

Pamela has received the Recognized Young Dietitian award for the state of Florida as well as the Award for Excellence in medical journalism by the Florida branch of the American Medical Association. She has been featured on radio and TV talk and news shows since 1980 and is in demand for corporate, top-management programs, seminars, conventions, and corporate wellness programs.